SpringerBriefs in Public Health

SpringerBriefs in Child Health

Series Editor
Angelo P. Giardino, Salt Lake City, UT, USA

SpringerBriefs in Public Health present concise summaries of cutting-edge research and practical applications from across the entire field of public health, with contributions from medicine, bioethics, health economics, public policy, biostatistics, and sociology.

The focus of the series is to highlight current topics in public health of interest to a global audience, including health care policy; social determinants of health; health issues in developing countries; new research methods; chronic and infectious disease epidemics; and innovative health interventions.

Featuring compact volumes of 50 to 125 pages, the series covers a range of content from professional to academic. Possible volumes in the series may consist of timely reports of state-of-the art analytical techniques, reports from the field, snapshots of hot and/or emerging topics, literature reviews, and in-depth case studies. Both solicited and unsolicited manuscripts are considered for publication in this series.

Briefs are published as part of Springer's eBook collection, with millions of users worldwide. In addition, Briefs are available for individual print and electronic purchase.

Briefs are characterized by fast, global electronic dissemination, standard publishing contracts, easy-to-use manuscript preparation and formatting guidelines, and expedited production schedules. We aim for publication 8–12 weeks after acceptance.

SpringerBriefs in Child Health present concise summaries of cutting-edge research and practical applications from the fields of child and adolescent health. This book series is designed to target children's health issues from birth through adolescence, from both a policy and practice perspective. Each subject in the series will be written by a specialist in that area. Their expertise will offer evaluation of the special health issues that would be of value to any health care provider. The authors all practice at nationally recognized children's hospitals and have done extensive research in their respective areas. The "template" for the series will be in three sections:

- "Snapshot from the Field" will address current practice and policy
- "Implications for Policy and Practice" will deal with the emerging science and best practices related to cutting edge work going on in the field
- "Looking Ahead" will look forward towards anticipated changes, recommendations and strategies to achieve the best for children and families.

Featuring compact volumes of 50 to 125 pages, the series covers a range of content from professional to academic. Possible volumes in the series may consist of timely reports of state-of-the-art analytical techniques, reports from the field, snapshots of hot and/or emerging topics, elaborated theses, literature reviews, and in-depth case studies. Both solicited and unsolicited manuscripts are considered for publication in this series. Briefs are published as part of Springer's eBook collection, with millions of users worldwide. In addition, Briefs are available for individual print and electronic purchase. Briefs are characterized by fast, global electronic dissemination, standard publishing contracts, easy-to-use manuscript preparation and formatting guidelines, and expedited production schedules. We aim for publication 8-12 weeks after acceptance.

Adam W. Dell • Jessica Robnett
Dana N. Johns • Emily M. Graham
Cori A. Agarwal • Lindsey Imber
Nicole L. Mihalopoulos

Providing Affirming Care to Transgender and Gender-Diverse Youth

With Contributions by Brett Myers
and Hayley McLaughlin

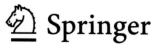 Springer

Adam W. Dell
Division of Adolescent Medicine,
Department of Pediatrics,
University of Utah
Salt Lake City, UT, USA

Dana N. Johns
Division of Plastic Surgery, Department
of Surgery
University of Utah
Salt Lake City, UT, USA

Cori A. Agarwal
Division of Plastic Surgery, Department
of Surgery
University of Utah
Salt Lake City, UT, USA

Nicole L. Mihalopoulos
Division of Adolescent Medicine,
Department of Pediatrics
University of Utah
Salt Lake City, UT, USA

Jessica Robnett
Division of Behavioral Health, Department
of Pediatrics
University of Utah
Salt Lake City, UT, USA

Emily M. Graham
Spencer Fox Eccles School of Medicine
University of Utah
Salt Lake City, UT, USA

Lindsey Imber
Communication Sciences and Disorders
University of Utah
Salt Lake City, UT, USA

Nutrition Care Services
University of Utah
Salt Lake City, UT, USA

ISSN 2192-3698   ISSN 2192-3701   (electronic)
SpringerBriefs in Public Health
ISSN 2625-2872   ISSN 2625-2880   (electronic)
SpringerBriefs in Child Health
ISBN 978-3-031-18454-3   ISBN 978-3-031-18455-0   (eBook)
https://doi.org/10.1007/978-3-031-18455-0

This Springer imprint is published by the registered company Springer Nature Switzerland AG
The registered company address is: Gewerbestrasse 11, 6330 Cham, Switzerland

Foreword

The authors of this monograph have produced a succinct, easy-to-read synthesis of the current understanding of how best to support youth and their families who are dealing with gender issues in the healthcare context. In 2018, the American Academy of Pediatrics (AAP) published a policy statement entitled, "Ensuring Comprehensive Care and Support for Transgender and Gender Diverse Children and Adolescents," which recognized that pediatric providers often have an essential role in assisting youth and families with gender concerns and in providing evidence-based information related to health and healthcare decisions (Rafferty et al. 2018). What we know, as stated in a healthychildren.org discussion of the AAP's gender-related policy statement, is that while transgender and gender-diverse children may face a number of challenges, they, like all children and youth, do best when they are supported and loved by those around them as they develop and grow into adulthood (AAP 2018). While being supportive of children and youth as they grow and develop may seem like common sense, all too often this caring approach to children and youth dealing with gender-related issues is not always present in their community environment. The 2018 AAP statement and this monograph adopt a gender-affirming care model (GACM) that, at its core, provides developmentally appropriate care that seeks to help youth and their families in gaining an understanding and appreciation for the youth's gender experience. Unlike the discredited conversion or reparative models of yesteryear, GACMs treat transgender youth as whole human beings who are developing and need support rather than discrimination and stigmatization. In large part, if mental disorders are identified in these youth, they tend to be as a result of responses to stigma or other negative experiences to which they are exposed rather than being intrinsic to the youth. Additionally, family acceptance or rejection "…may profoundly affect young people's ability to openly discuss or disclose concerns about their identity" and "suppressing such concerns can affect mental health" (Rafferty et al. 2018, p. 8). With this in mind, clinicians and policymakers, as well as those interested in learning more about current best practices related to gender-affirming care, will find this monograph useful as an introduction into how best to offer support to youth and families in the pediatric healthcare setting.

Pediatrics is defined as the specialty in medicine concerned with addressing the physical, mental, and social health of children from birth to young adulthood (American Academy of Pediatrics Committee on Pediatric Workforce et al. 2015). Of note, the definition is oriented toward serving all children and makes no distinction about which populations of children and families are included or those who should be excluded. Pediatric health care is at its best when those providing the care approach youth and families with respect for the youth's experiences and with a sense of commitment toward promoting the physical, mental, and social health needs of that specific patient and their family. What will become clear after reading this monograph is that those who seek to address the healthcare needs of transgender and gender-diverse youth provide optimal care by adopting a supportive and affirming approach grounded in a care environment that fosters dialogue and exploration of the many issues that may be present. Sadly, this supportive and affirming approach to care for these youth and their families has not always been readily available. Now, with an increasing focus and an emerging evidence base, pediatric and child-serving professionals can be better equipped to facilitate developmentally appropriate dialogue with youth and families around transgender and gender-diverse experiences. One of the foundational principles of ethical medical practice, included in the Hippocratic Oath, is the notion of "first, do no harm." In line with this "do no harm" principle, a worthy goal is to be welcoming to all youth and their families, including those who are dealing with gender issues, and to seek to contribute in a positive and constructive way to their achieving maximal health and well-being. The clinical approach described in this monograph is firmly rooted in this inclusive attitude toward providing pediatric care. The authors provide a stepwise, coherent method on how best to deliver care that is consistent with a gender-affirming model. Meeting the youth where they are and helping them and their families make sense of their experiences with the goal of achieving optimal health and well-being are ultimately just part of delivering ideal pediatric care to those we have the privilege of serving as healthcare providers.

Salt Lake City, UT, USA   Angelo P. Giardino, MD, PhD

References

American Academy of Pediatrics (2018) AAP policy statement urges support and care of transgender and gender-diverse children and adolescents. https://www.healthychildren.org. Accessed 24 Feb 2022

American Academy of Pediatrics Committee on Pediatric Workforce, Rimsza ME, Hotaling AJ, Keown ME, Marcin JP, Moskowitz WB, et al. (2015) Definition of a pediatrician. Pediatrics 135(4):780–781. https://doi.org/10.1542/peds.2015-0056

Committee on Psychosocial Aspects of Child and Family Health, Committee on Adolescence, & Section on Lesbian, Gay, Bisexual, and Transgender Health and Wellness Rafferty J, (2018) Ensuring comprehensive care and support for transgender and gender-diverse children and adolescents. Pediatrics 142(4):e20182162. https://doi.org/10.1542/peds.2018-2162

Contents

About the Authors

Adam W. Dell, MD, is a board-certified pediatrician and adolescent medicine provider at the University of Utah. His clinical interests include primary care for underrepresented groups, including indigenous populations and LGBTQI youth. He enjoys providing gender-affirming care and mental health services to gender-diverse youth. He is an enrolled member of the Pine Ridge Indian Reservation. He completed a residency in pediatrics at the University of Utah. His research interests include expanding diversity, inclusion, and equity to resident education; bridging the gap between gender-affirming care and primary care; and physician wellness. Dr. Dell feels that as healthcare providers, gender diversity needs to be more than accepted—it needs to be celebrated. It is his passion to help train more general pediatricians to be gender-affirming champions.

Jessica Robnett, PsyD, received her PsyD in Clinical Psychology from the Georgia School of Professional Psychology at Argosy University with practicum training at Children's Healthcare of Atlanta. She completed her internship at Miami Children's Hospital and postdoctoral fellowship at Primary Children's Hospital, specializing in Pediatric Psychology. Dr. Robnett is a visiting assistant professor of Pediatrics at the University of Utah School of Medicine and is in the Division of Pediatric Behavioral Health. Her primary clinical interests include the assessment and treatment of children and adolescents with medical illnesses with work in both pulmonology and adolescent medicine. Her research interests include mental health in pediatric cystic fibrosis patients and integration of behavioral health services into subspecialty clinics.

Dana N. Johns, MD, is a board-certified plastic surgeon at the University of Utah and specializes in all areas of craniofacial surgery, including cleft lip, nose and palate deformities, craniosynostosis, ear reconstruction and posttraumatic reconstruction, and facial feminization, as well as general pediatric plastic surgery. Her clinical interests also include facial cosmetic surgery and gender confirmation surgery. She is a native of Pennsylvania and earned her undergraduate degree from Franklin and Marshall College and her medical degree from Thomas Jefferson Medical College. She completed a Plastic and Reconstructive Surgery Residency at the University of Utah and a Cleft and Craniofacial Fellowship at Stanford University. Dr. Johns enjoys spending her free time with her family and is an avid rock climber, snowboarder, and oil painter.

Emily M. Graham, BSN, is a medical student at the University of Utah. Prior to matriculating into medical school, Emily worked as a nurse, where she developed a passion for patient advocacy and reconstructive surgery. Emily hopes to enrich her patients' lives through clinical care, research, and continued advocacy.

Cori A. Agarwal, MD, is a board-certified plastic surgeon at the University of Utah. She is originally from the Big Island of Hawaii. After graduating from Yale University, she attended medical school at the University of Hawaii John A. Burns School of Medicine. She completed her residency in General Surgery and Plastic Surgery at the University of Chicago followed by a fellowship year with Dr. Jack Owsley at the California Medical Center in San Francisco. She is the cofounder and medical director of the University of Utah Transgender Multidisciplinary Health Program and has a busy practice in gender-affirming surgery. Dr. Agarwal performs a range of gender-affirming surgeries and is recognized as a leader and an expert in the area of chest masculinization. She has published and presented extensively on the subject, specifically in the areas of quality of life improvement, patient-reported outcomes, and surgical technique.

Lindsey Imber, MS, RD, CD, is a classically trained chef who studied culinary arts at Johnson and Wales University. After nearly a decade of working in restaurants and cooking for sports teams, she wanted to figure out how she could use her love of food to help people. She has since received her graduate degree in Nutrition and Integrative Physiology from the University of Utah and has worked as a clinical dietitian since 2018. She spent three years with the Adolescent Medicine Clinic at the University of Utah working with transgender and gender-diverse adolescents. She is currently the Patient Services Manager for HCA Healthcare at St. Mark's hospital. Through her passion for food and knowledge of nutrition, she is able to help patients find happiness and health in every bite of food they take.

Nicole L. Mihalopoulos, MD, MPH, is a board-certified adolescent medicine physician and Chief of the Division of Adolescent Medicine in the Department of Pediatrics at the University of Utah. She is the founder and medical director of the University of Utah Health Adolescent Medicine Clinic and the Primary Children's Hospital Gender Management and Support (GeMS) Clinic. These clinics comprise a multidisciplinary team of providers including Adolescent Medicine, Adolescent Psychology, Registered Dietitian, and Nurse Coordinator. She is board certified in Internal Medicine, Preventive Medicine, and Adolescent Medicine. As a clinician scientist, her research focuses on cardiovascular disease risk factors among adolescents.

About the Contributors

Hayley McLaughlin, RN, has worked as a registered nurse in the Adolescent Medicine Clinic at the University of Utah for three years, assisting in the coordination of patient care and management of the clinic. She is passionate about the emotional and physical health of adolescents, young adults, and the families that love and support them, both at work and in life.

Brett Myers, PhD, CCC-SLP, is an assistant professor in the Department of Communication Sciences and Disorders at the University of Utah. He completed a BA in Psychology and Voice and Speech at McDaniel College, an MA in Communication Sciences and Disorders at the University of Iowa, and a PhD in Interdisciplinary Studies: Hearing and Speech and Psychology at Vanderbilt University.Dr. Myers is the Interim Director of Clinical Education in Speech-Language Pathology at the University of Utah. He instructs and supervises graduate students in conducting behavioral treatment of voice disorders. Additionally, Dr. Myers serves as Digital Associate Editor for the Psychonomic Society. Dr. Myers' research interests include cognitive processes in speech production, motor control of voice and speech, and treatment modalities in voice disorders.

Chapter 1
Introduction

Adam W. Dell

Terms and Definition

Sexuality and gender identity are independent terms that are often classified together. Sexuality refers to the sexual orientation or sexual attraction behaviors of an individual, while gender identity refers to the intrinsic sense of one's gender. Table 1.1 provides definitions of terms describing sexuality and gender identity.

Population Trends

Assignment of an individual's sex (male, female, intersex) is generally made at birth based on anatomy and, for some, on chromosomal analysis. This assignment will help mold gender identity (the innate sense of maleness or femaleness) as the individual matures (Hembree et al. 2017). Gender identity is a social construct. Some individuals' gender identities will differ from their assigned birth sex, resulting from a combination of social, biological, cultural, and environmental factors (Rosenthal 2016; Wylie et al. 2016). These individuals may be regarded as gender diverse or transgender.

An estimated 0.6% of adults (approximately 1.4 million) in the United States identify as transgender (The Williams Institute 2017). The Williams Institute uses Behavioral Risk Factor Surveillance System data to estimate the percentage of adults who identify as transgender in the United States. Estimating the prevalence

A. W. Dell (✉)
Division of Adolescent Medicine, Department of Pediatrics, University of Utah,
Salt Lake City, UT, USA
e-mail: adam.dell@hsc.utah.edu

© The Author(s), under exclusive license to Springer Nature Switzerland AG 2022
A. W. Dell et al., *Providing Affirming Care to Transgender and Gender-Diverse Youth*, SpringerBriefs in Public Health, https://doi.org/10.1007/978-3-031-18455-0_1

Table 1.1 Definition of terms describing sexuality and gender identity

Term	Definition
Asexual	Not experiencing sexual attraction
Assigned sex at birth/birth sex/natal sex	The sex assigned to a person at birth by their healthcare team, usually based on genital anatomy, occasionally using genetics
Bisexual	Sexual attraction to males and females
Cisgender	Having a gender identity that corresponds to one's sex as assigned at birth
Gender diverse/gender expansive/gender non-conforming	Having a gender identity or gender expression that does not conform to or expands beyond socially defined male/female gender norms
Gender dysphoria	The emotional discomfort experienced by people whose gender does not align with their sex as assigned at birth
Genderfluid	Sense of gender fluctuates between feminine and masculine
Genderqueer	Sense of gender identity differs from sex as assigned at birth, but is not in the transgender binary (transmale or transfemale)
Intersex/disorders of sex development	Having sex chromosomes that differ from external or internal reproductive anatomy
Legal sex	The gender marker that appears on government issued identification documents
Non-binary gender	Identifying as neither female/feminine nor male/masculine
Pansexual	Sexual attraction toward all sex/gender identities
Preferred gender	The gender (boy/man or girl/woman) an individual self-identifies as, often through outward presentation (clothing, hair) and chosen name and pronouns
Sexuality	Sexual attraction toward a specific sex or gender
Social transition	The fully reversible process of gender presentation through clothing, body shapers, body language, hair, name, pronouns
Transfemale/transfeminine/transwoman/transgirl	A person who identifies as female (woman/girl) and was assigned male at birth (typically having male genitalia at birth)
Transgender	Having a gender identity that is opposite of one's sex as assigned at birth
Transmale/transmasculine/transman/transboy	A person who identifies as male (man/boy) and was assigned female at birth (typically having female genitalia at birth)

of children and adolescents who are transgender was very difficult prior to 2017 because many states did not collect the needed data. For example, the Utah Department of Health included questions about sexuality and gender identity on the Utah Youth Risk Behavior Survey for the first time in 2019 (Utah Department of Health 2019). A recent study using data from 19 states reported that 1.8% of youth identified as transgender (Johns et al. 2019). This report only included people who identify as transgender and did not include people who are gender diverse (non-binary, genderqueer, genderfluid) and identify as other than transgender or cisgender.

Awareness and Acceptance

In January 2017, National Geographic released a special issue titled, "Gender Revolution: The Shifting Landscape of Gender" (2017). Gender diversity is not a revolution at all. Gender diversity has been present in many cultures, including indigenous cultures, for centuries. Many of these cultures identify gender diversity as a normal human variant of an individual's identity. Unfortunately, in other cultures, gender diversity is a foreign topic that promotes a sense of discomfort due to a lack of understanding.

Transgender and gender-diverse visibility has been on the rise in media, schools, and public policy. This is likely due to increasing awareness and slow acceptance of gender-diverse individuals. Social media may also play a role in increasing awareness of gender diversity. More children and young adults are defining their identities in diverse ways. Unfortunately, society's discomfort with nonconformity promotes unique challenges to gender-diverse individuals due to a lack of understanding, feeling as though gender diversity is "abnormal," or regarding gender diversity as unnatural. It is difficult for some to get away from a binary way of thinking—that a person is either a man or a woman with no in-between. There is also a poor understanding that sex assigned at birth, gender identity, and sexual identity do not have to be in relation to each other. They are three completely different components of a person's identity. In the absence of universal acceptance, many gender-diverse individuals struggle with discrimination, minority stress, poor access to health care, mental health disparities, and other inequities.

Gender Dysphoria

Many people who are transgender or gender diverse may experience gender dysphoria, the intense emotional distress that is caused by a "discrepancy between a person's gender identity and that person's sex assigned at birth" (World Professional Association for Transgender Health 2022, p. 5). Gender dysphoria may present as emotional withdrawal, problems at school, self-harm, and suicidality. Gender dysphoria can be mitigated with supportive and affirming families and social networks, and, in some, gender-affirming medical treatment, and for fewer, surgical treatment. It is often addressed through several domains, including:

- Social

    - Use of the individual's affirmed name
    - Use of the individual's affirmed pronouns
    - Affirming gender presentation (congruent clothing, behaviors, expression, use of bathrooms)

- Psychological
  - Sense of authentic self-identity
  - Mental healthcare from providers who are knowledgeable about gender-focused therapy and the needs of transgender individuals. These providers can help define goals of medical care as well as address internalized transphobia, depression, and anxiety.

- Medical
  - Gender-affirming hormones that are safely managed
  - Sexual health considerations, including contraception and fertility preservation
  - Primary care from clinicians familiar with the needs of transgender individuals
  - Gender-affirming surgeries and procedures
  - Voice and communication therapies

- Legal
  - Effective anti-discrimination legislation
  - Access to legal providers
  - Legal name change and change of gender designation
  - Right to recognition under the law (Winter et al. 2016; Wylie et al. 2016)

Gender-Affirming Care

With the increased awareness of gender diversity, there must also be an increase in understanding and competency so that this population can feel safe and affirmed in settings of school, work, and the doctor's office (Wylie et al. 2016). Healthcare institutions must change the way they care for gender-diverse individuals by providing affirming access to care, utilizing appropriate identification information including affirmed name/pronouns, formatting their forms and electronic medical record to accommodate affirming language, educating providers and support staff, and advocating for the unique needs of gender-diverse people.

Many professional societies support the provision of gender-affirming care to gender-diverse youth (Lopez et al. 2017; Society for Adolescent Health and Medicine 2013; Hembree et al. 2017; Rafferty et al. 2018). In 2018, the American Academy of Pediatrics (AAP) issued a policy statement promoting the support and care of transgender and gender-diverse youth focusing on gender-affirming and nonjudgmental approaches when caring for this population (Rafferty et al. 2018). The AAP recommends:

- Providing youth with access to comprehensive gender-affirming and developmentally appropriate health care
- Providing family-based therapy and support to meet the needs of parents, caregivers, and siblings of youth who identify as transgender
- Assuring that electronic health records, billing systems, patient-centered notification systems, and clinical research are designed to respect the asserted gender identity of each patient while maintaining confidentiality

- Supporting insurance plans that offer coverage specific to the needs of youth who identify as transgender, including coverage for medical, psychological, and, when appropriate, surgical interventions (Rafferty et al. 2018)

Professional medical societies must continue to advocate for the needs of this population as more research must be done to understand the long-term risks and benefits of gender-affirming medical care. Societies must also advocate against harmful laws that may affect access to care and human rights. Laws must be enacted to protect the physical and psychological safety of this population. Overall, we must stop looking at gender diversity as a problem. We must regard gender diversity as a normal variant of human nature.

References

Hembree WC, Cohen-Kettenis PT, Gooren L et al (2017) Endocrine treatment of gender-dysphoric/gender-incongruent persons: an endocrine society clinical practice guideline. J Clin Endocrinol Metab 102(11):3869–3903. https://doi.org/10.1210/jc.2017-01658

Johns MM, Lowry R, Andrzejewski J et al (2019) Transgender identity and experiences of violence victimization, substance use, suicide risk, and sexual risk behaviors among high school students - 19 states and large urban school districts, 2017. MMWR Morb Mortal Wkly Rep 68(3):67–71. https://doi.org/10.15585/mmwr.mm6803a3

Lopez X, Marinkovic M, Eimicke T et al (2017) Statement on gender-affirmative approach to care from the pediatric endocrine society special interest group on transgender health. Curr Opin Pediatr 29(4):475–480. https://doi.org/10.1097/MOP.0000000000000516

National Geographic Society (2017) Special issue: gender revolution – the shifting landscape of gender. National Geographic 1 Jan 2017:1–154

Rafferty J, Committee on Psychosocial Aspects of Child and Family Health, Committee on Adolescence, Section on Lesbian, Gay, Bisexual, And Transgender Health and Wellness (2018) Ensuring comprehensive care and support for transgender and gender-diverse children and adolescents. Pediatrics 142(4):e20182162. https://doi.org/10.1542/peds.2018-2162

Rosenthal SM (2016) Transgender youth: current concepts. Ann Pediatr Endocrinol Metab 21(4):185–192. https://doi.org/10.6065/apem.2016.21.4.185

Society for Adolescent Health and Medicine (2013) Recommendations for promoting the health and well-being of lesbian, gay, bisexual, and transgender adolescents: a position paper of the Society for Adolescent Health and Medicine. J Adolesc Health 52(4):506–510. https://doi.org/10.1016/j.jadohealth.2013.01.015

The Williams Institute (2017) Transgender people. https://williamsinstitute.law.ucla.edu/subpopulations/transgender-people/. Accessed 6 Apr 2021

Utah Department of Health (2019) 2019 behavioral risk factor surveillance system questionnaire. In: BRFSS data in action current and past questionnaires. Center for Health Data and Informatics, Office of Public Health Assessment. https://opha.health.utah.gov/access-brfss-data/. Accessed 5 Oct 2020

Winter S, Diamond M, Green J et al (2016) Transgender people: health at the margins of society. Lancet 388(10042):390–400. https://doi.org/10.1016/S0140-6736(16)00683-8

World Professional Association for Transgender Health (WPATH) (2022) Standards of care for the health of transgender and gender diverse people, version 8. https://www.wpath.org/publications/soc

Wylie K, Knudson G, Khan SI et al (2016) Serving transgender people: clinical care considerations and service delivery models in transgender health. Lancet 388(10042):401–411. https://doi.org/10.1016/S0140-6736(16)00682-6

Chapter 2
Identity Development and Mental Health

Jessica Robnett

Introduction

As awareness and visibility of transgender adolescents increases, along with related social/political controversy, the need to recognize and address their challenges and support their mental health has become more urgent. Understanding the development of gender and sexual identity and the potential impacts of nonconformity in these areas on mental health is key for clinicians. Optimal approaches to mental health care are evolving, though lack of trained clinicians limits access.

Adolescent health care is complicated due to the importance of having productive interactions with both the teen and their caregiver(s). Ideally, the clinician has the opportunity to meet individually with all parties to better understand the overall goals, expectations, and concerns related to care. The clinician's role entails listening to the patient and hearing their deep concerns, not just the surface-level complaints, and then partnering with the patient to come up with a plan to keep them safe and healthy, both physically and emotionally. For adolescents, it is imperative that this plan includes their "safe people"—parents, legal guardians, or whoever provides them support.

Identity Development

The presentation of gender diversity in children and adolescents appears to be highly bimodal. There are individuals who, in their early development, recognize that the sex assigned to them at birth does not fit their experience of themselves.

J. Robnett (✉)
Division of Behavioral Health, Department of Pediatrics, University of Utah,
Salt Lake City, UT, USA
e-mail: mountainpedpsych@gmail.com

© The Author(s), under exclusive license to Springer Nature Switzerland AG 2022
A. W. Dell et al., *Providing Affirming Care to Transgender and Gender-Diverse Youth*, SpringerBriefs in Public Health, https://doi.org/10.1007/978-3-031-18455-0_2

These are often young children who are adamant that they were given the wrong body. There are also individuals who begin to question their identity as potentially unwelcome changes occur during puberty. In early childhood, strangers often assign a gender label based on appearance of hair, clothing, and behaviors, but non-conforming children are often given leeway to explore their own expression. Society is much less kind to those with visible secondary sex characteristics that do not conform. When an adolescent's body starts to change in ways that are discordant with their gender identity, it can trigger a strong dysphoria. (See Chap. 1 for definition of gender dysphoria.)

Early Childhood

Identity development is an ongoing process that starts in early childhood and continues across one's life. Early childhood is a time of exploration and trying to make sense of the world. Naming or labeling objects, places, and people (and their characteristics) helps children find rules to guide their understanding of the world and their experiences. In early childhood, children recognize their race, gender, and family structures. They notice, and often say something, when things don't "feel right."

As early as age 2 or 3, most children can label their own assigned gender. By age 4, they understand that gender is stable over time, and by age 6, children understand that gender is consistent across situations. For example, they know that a boy will not become a girl by wearing a dress or playing with dolls (Kohlberg 1966).

Exploration of gender-normative expectations is part of figuring out the rules of the world. Children want to know why something is a "girl thing" or a "boy thing." Many children at this age will express gender diversity and question if the label they've been assigned fits who they are. In research, male-assigned children more often present with variance and questioning in childhood than those who are assigned female, with reports as high as 3, or even 6, birth-assigned males for each birth-assigned female (Zucker 2004). This raises questions about the rigidity of society's rules for each of these groups. One theory is that females are typically allowed much more flexibility in their interests than males (e.g., both boys and girls in our society can play with trucks, but boys' interest in dolls is less accepted).

Two studies have addressed persistence of gender variance in children. A 2019 study included 84 children under the age of 12 who presented with gender diversity but had not socially transitioned. After 2 years, 41% of these children had socially transitioned to their identified gender; greater dysphoria on initial contact correlated with increased likelihood of persistence (Rae et al. 2019). A longitudinal study published in 2022 examined re-transition rates of 317 transgender children initially between ages 3 and 12 who had "completed" a binary transition. At 5-year follow-up, 94% of these individuals identified as binary transgender, 3.5% identified as non-binary, and only 2.5% identified as cisgender (Olsen et al. 2022). This very important finding demonstrates that identity in childhood after social transition is generally quite stable.

Puberty

Adolescence is a time of significant identity exploration and change. Developmental theorists say it is a period of separating from one's family and further exploring individual wants and needs. Peers become drivers of exploration, providing exposure to different ideas and ways of thinking and being. Additionally, physical changes of puberty can create dissonance for adolescents who previously weren't "that bothered" by societal norms associated with their assigned birth gender. These physical changes can trigger significant dysphoria in adolescents whose emerging gender identity diverges from the one they've lived with to date.

It is not uncommon for individuals with no prior history of gender nonconformity to present with new onset gender dysphoria in adolescence. Though research is limited, it is believed that the gender identity of adolescents presenting with gender dysphoria is likely to persist into adulthood. One clinic reported that of 70 adolescents who presented with gender dysphoria in adolescence, all persisted and started gender-affirming hormones (de Vries et al. 2011). A review of the ten available prospective studies of children with gender dysphoria followed to adolescence reported that about 20% experience persistence of gender dysphoria (Ristori and Steensma 2016).

The CDC currently estimates that 2% of current high school students identify as transgender (Johns et al. 2019). Limited prevalence studies suggest that in adolescence, unlike in younger children, gender dysphoria is distributed much more equally across those assigned male and female at birth (1:1) (Cohen-Kettenis and Pfafflin 2003). However, the patient population at the University of Utah Adolescent Medicine Clinic is skewed, with 70% assigned female at birth.

Gender Isn't Just "Boy" and "Girl": Acknowledging and Supporting All Identities

As we support those who are born into a gender-incongruent body, it is important to recognize that our traditional polarization of gender into male and female is quite limiting. Some individuals find that their experience of gender equally encompasses both masculine and feminine, or maybe they don't feel that either a masculine or feminine identity fits. Regardless of how a person identifies, it is important to respect their experience, their pronouns, and their name. Even those who identify as transgender may wish to be "stealth" or not share their identity journey with others. Some will choose to have one or many surgeries to affirm their gender, others will choose only to change their hair, makeup, and clothing style (gender expression), and some will change nothing external at all. A person's journey and experience of themselves is uniquely individual. The best outcomes for gender-diverse children and adolescents are achieved through supporting them as unique individuals and helping them address the numerous challenges they may face to becoming the healthiest versions of themselves.

Gender Diversity Is Not a Mental Health Diagnosis

Gender diversity, or not matching gender norms or stereotypes, is not considered a mental health diagnosis. To meet criteria for a mental health diagnosis, there must be a key element of distress or impairment in functioning. Not all individuals who are gender diverse experience distress or impairment related to their identity. The DSM-5 (American Psychiatric Association [APA] 2013) currently provides criteria for diagnosing gender dysphoria, but gender diversity is not, and should not, be pathologized.

When present, gender dysphoria can be treated with both medical and mental health interventions.

"Well-Controlled" Mental Health: Anxiety and Depression

Adolescents that identify as transgender have significantly higher rates of depression compared to their cisgender peers, with as many as 66% of individuals reporting related symptoms (APA 2013). They also have higher rates of suicidal ideation, plans, and attempts (Thoma et al. 2019). The role of the gender health team is to support a person's health and development. This may include medications to suppress or initiate hormonal effects, emotional support, support for healthy eating, and voice training.

The Role of Mental Health Professionals

In this journey, there are crucial decisions that children, adolescents, and their families may have to make. Starting puberty blockers, affirming hormones, and surgical interventions are generally why patients present to a medical clinic, but understanding a patient's social and emotional supports is important as well. The mental health professional's goal is generally to ensure that the patient has the skills and supports to thrive during their transition and beyond. Within the World Professional Association for Transgender Health (WPATH) standards of care, the role of a mental health professional includes assessment of the patient's understanding and expectations of their desired medical care (WPATH 2022). Unrealistic expectations can be very harmful in terms of mental health. It is important that patients recognize the time that medicines take to reach full effect. The role of a mental health professional is not to be a "gatekeeper" but rather to identify and provide support in overcoming barriers to thriving. Appropriate assessment, diagnosis, and treatment of existing mental health concerns help provide a more stable base for the changes that occur when undergoing gender-affirming treatment. Mental health treatment may focus on developing skills to better manage anxiety or depression, improve self-esteem, and improve social skills or on helping an adolescent's support system navigate their decision making. Of note, "treatment" intended to change a person's gender identity or expression has proven to be unsuccessful and is unethical and harmful.

Case Study: A Parent's Perspective
Hayley McLaughlin

My name is Hayley, and I am mom to two adolescent boys, 19 and 16. When my youngest son was in the sixth and seventh grades, he was really struggling with school, friendships, and anxiety and depression. He was obsessed with makeup and social media and seemed to be one person online and another at home. Over the course of 2 years, he had not always been honest, and I found it difficult to trust him when he'd report his daily experiences. I wish I could say that he trusted me enough to come out to me, but in the end, it was his brother who told me that Alex was trans.

Ben and Alex were not close, not even a little bit, but one evening after another in a series of countless arguments between Alex and me, Ben sat beside me and said that Alex was a boy and probably wasn't eating because he didn't want his breasts to grow. When Alex came home minutes later, he realized his brother had outed him and explained that he "just didn't know how to tell me." Before the week was over, we had an appointment with a doctor to get Alex on a hormone blocker.

I can remember feeling like it was a matter of life or death at that point, as if I were trying to make up for the time lost while Alex tried to work this out without my support. I spent hours on the phone with our insurance company and specialty pharmacies to get medication and gender-affirming therapy for my child. I remember feeling relieved as I lined up therapy appointments, knowing his hormones were "paused" while he explored his gender identity. I worked hard to use male pronouns and his new name and discussed changes and expectations with his school and our family. Even though Alex was overwhelmingly supported after coming out, his issues with anxiety and depression did not seem to resolve. Alex spent the next 2 years working on issues related and unrelated to his gender identity.

Alex started testosterone at 14. After being eager to start hormones for the better part of 2 years, when he finally got the go-ahead from his therapist, family, and doctor, it was Alex that opted to wait another 6 months to make sure he was emotionally ready. About 4 months after starting testosterone, his voice had begun to change, and he began to carry himself in a way that seemed more confident and more himself. My parents commented that he laughed more and seemed more at ease with himself and in the world.

Now at 16, Alex has a job he likes, he feels good about school, and he has just had chest masculinization surgery. He doesn't report feeling anxiety and depression outside of what I'd expect from a teenager living in today's world.

(continued)

Case Study (continued)

Recently we discussed his transition, and I asked him when he knew he was trans. I shared a memory of him introducing himself as "Sam" in his kindergarten circle. He told me he didn't remember that day in school, and he denied any feeling of being any gender at all until puberty started. He reported feeling like it just wasn't him and feeling "wrong in my body" and not knowing how to articulate those feelings. As I reflect upon Alex's journey, the more I let him direct his own timing with his transition, the more he did the work he needed to do to make good choices for himself. I am inexpressibly grateful that we had access to medical care and therapy along every step of his journey; I shudder to think of what might have happened if we had not been able to get him on a hormone blocker, affirm his gender with hormone therapy, and have access to ongoing therapy and mental health support. I'm thankful, as well, to all the teachers, family, and friends that have supported Alex and me over the last 6 years; I certainly couldn't have been enough or done enough for Alex on my own. It takes community support to raise healthy and happy kids.

Gender Diversity and Autism Spectrum Disorder: Frequent Overlap?

Studies have suggested that the prevalence of gender variance in individuals with autism spectrum disorder (ASD) is 5–7% (de Vries et al. 2010), which is much higher than the general population where estimates are closer to 1% (Lai et al. 2014). A 2018 article in the *Journal of the American Academy of Child and Adolescent Psychiatry* challenged the criteria used to identify "gender variance" in those with ASD as not capturing dysphoria but rather a "wish to be the opposite sex" on a Likert scale (never, sometimes, or often) (Turban and van Schalkwyk 2018). Some children may transiently wish to be the opposite sex without having a true transgendered identity. It also challenged studies that took the opposite approach, using a screener for ASD in a population with gender dysphoria (Turban and van Schalkwyk 2018). These studies estimated that 6–10% of those with gender identity disorder (GID), a now unused diagnosis that has been replaced by gender dysphoria, have comorbid ASD (de Vries et al. 2010), with as many as 45% of individuals having clinical traits of ASD (VanderLaan et al. 2015). Turban and van Schalkwyk (2018) countered that social impairments could be the result of experiences that youth with gender dysphoria face rather than true, underlying ASD. They concluded that it is important to recognize that people with ASD experience a spectrum of gender and, likewise, recognize that individuals with gender dysphoria may have more difficulties with typical social interactions (Turban and van Schalkwyk 2018).

Disparities in Access

In most cases, minors are dependent on their parents or guardians for access to medical care. In some states, adolescents have individual rights around sexual or mental health care, but our traditional healthcare system is set up to require parental consent for medical intervention. In addition, even those who are able to consent to their own treatment are unable to access their own insurance or financial resources for care. This creates a significant barrier for individuals whose guardians do not support gender-affirming medical transition.

However, even patients with affirming and supportive caregivers may face significant barriers in accessing appropriate medical care. This can be due to lack of knowledgeable medical providers, being uninsured or underinsured, housing problems, lack of adequate transportation, and/or food insecurity.

Accessing gender-affirming care has recently become politicized, and a battle is raging in state legislatures regarding the ability of clinicians to provide and families to seek life-saving medical care for adolescents.

Acknowledgments The author thanks Hayley McLaughlin, RN, for the contribution to Chap. 2.

References

American Psychiatric Association (APA) (2013) Diagnostic and statistical manual of mental disorders fifth edition (DSM-5). American Psychiatric Association Publishing, Washington, D.C.

Cohen-Kettenis PT, Pfafflin F (2003) Transgenderism and intersexuality in childhood and adolescence: making choices. Sage Publications, Thousand Oaks

de Vries AL, Noens IL, Cohen-Kettenis PT et al (2010) Autism spectrum disorders in gender dysphoric children and adolescents. J Autism Dev Disord 40(8):930–936. https://doi.org/10.1007/s10803-010-0935-9

de Vries AL, Steensma TD, Doreleijers TA et al (2011) Puberty suppression in adolescents with gender identity disorder: a prospective follow-up study. J Sex Med 8(8):2276–2283. https://doi.org/10.1111/j.1743-6109.2010.01943.x

Johns MM, Lowry R, Andrzejewski J et al (2019) Transgender identity and experiences of violence victimization, substance abuse, suicide risk, and sexual risk behaviors among high school students – 19 states and large urban school districts, 2017. Morb Mortal Wkly Rep 68:67–71. https://doi.org/10.15585/mmwr.mm6803a3

Kohlberg L (1966) A cognitive-developmental analysis of children's sex-role concepts and attitudes. In: Maccoby EE (ed) The development of sex differences. Stanford University Press, Stanford, pp 82–173

Lai MD, Lombardo MV, Baron-Cohen S (2014) Autism. Lancet 383:896–910

Olson KR, Durwood L, Horton R et al (2022) Gender identity 5 years after social transition. Pediatrics 150. https://doi.org/10.1542/peds.2021-056082

Rae JR, Gülgöz S, Durwood L et al (2019) Predicting early-childhood gender transitions. Psychol Sci 30(5):669–681. https://doi.org/10.1177/0956797619830649

Ristori J, Steensma TD (2016) Gender dysphoria in childhood. Int Rev Psychiatry 28(1):13–20. https://doi.org/10.3109/09540261.2015.1115754

Thoma BC, Salk RH, Choukas-Bradley S et al (2019) Suicidality disparities between transgender and cisgender adolescents. Pediatrics 144(5):e20191183. https://doi.org/10.1542/peds.2019-1183

Turban JL, van Schalkwyk GI (2018) "Gender dysphoria" and autism spectrum disorder: is the link real? J Am Acad Child Adolesc Psychiatry 57(1):8–9. https://doi.org/10.1016/j.jaac.2017.08.017

VanderLaan DP, Leef JH, Wood H et al (2015) Autism spectrum disorder risk factors and autistic traits in gender dysphoric children. J Autism Dev Disord 45(6):1742–1750. https://doi.org/10.1007/s10803-014-2331-3

World Professional Association for Transgender Health (WPATH) (2022) Standards of care for the health of transgender and gender diverse people, version 8. https://www.wpath.org/publications/soc

Zucker KJ (2004) Gender identity development and issues. Child Adolesc Psychiatr Clin N Am 13(3):551–568. https://doi.org/10.1016/j.chc.2004.02.006

Chapter 3
Gender Affirmation: Medical

Adam W. Dell

Introduction

Using gender-affirming medications to address gender dysphoria in adolescents is a shared medical decision between the patient, the patient's parents/legal guardians, and the physician (see Chap. 1 for definition of gender dysphoria). Currently, many providers choose to integrate guidelines proposed by the Endocrine Society and the World Professional Association for Transgender Health (World Professional Association for Transgender Health [WPATH] 2022). There are a variety of medical treatment options available to patients based on gender identity, goals of care, stage of pubertal development, and comfort of family members providing consent for care. Determining what therapies are appropriate also depends on the patient's goals and where they are on their gender journey. While some patients may not desire any medical interventions, others regard these therapies as necessary and lifesaving.

Background and History

Much of our knowledge regarding the use of gender-affirming medications in this population comes from over 30 years of clinical observation in the Netherlands. "The Dutch Model" was published in 2006 (Delemarre-van de Waal and Cohen-Kettenis 2006), outlining the use of puberty blockers (gonadotropin-releasing hormone [GnRH] analogues) at the age of 12 and the initiation of gender-affirming

A. W. Dell (✉)
Division of Adolescent Medicine, Department of Pediatrics, University of Utah,
Salt Lake City, UT, USA
e-mail: e-mail: adam.dell@hsc.utah.edu

© The Author(s), under exclusive license to Springer Nature Switzerland AG 2022
A. W. Dell et al., *Providing Affirming Care to Transgender and Gender-Diverse Youth*, SpringerBriefs in Public Health, https://doi.org/10.1007/978-3-031-18455-0_3

hormones (testosterone and estrogen) at the age of 16. One of the biggest limitations of this model is the focus on chronologic age. Many individuals experience an onset of puberty well before the age of 12. Furthermore, requiring a patient to wait until the age of 16 to experience desired secondary sex characteristics while their peers are experiencing puberty is also problematic. To address this issue, The Endocrine Society published clinical guidelines, "Endocrine Treatment of Transexual Persons," which were then updated in 2017 (Hembree et al. 2009, 2017). The guidelines focus on the idea that puberty blockers are to be initiated based on the patient's development of secondary sex characteristics and that induction of gender-affirming puberty may be carefully explored in patients before the age of 16.

Puberty Blockers

Puberty blockers are traditionally used at the onset of puberty, around sexual maturity (formerly "Tanner") stages 2 or 3. For many, the development of undesired secondary sex characteristics is distressing. This promotes further gender incongruence that exacerbates gender dysphoria. Puberty blockers attempt to address this issue by putting a temporal pause on further progress of the undesired puberty. This can allow for more time for gender exploration. For transmasculine individuals, the use of puberty blockers may prevent the need for chest masculinizing surgery later in life and prevents the development of a gynecoid pelvis. For transfeminine individuals, puberty blockers prevent the deepening of the voice and progression of irreversible masculine body features (facial hair, broader shoulders, and larger hands and feet). Much of our knowledge of puberty blockers comes from their use to treat precocious puberty in the pediatric population.

Traditionally, GnRH analogues in the form of an injection or an implantable subcutaneous rod are used. The decision to use these medications is often limited by their cost as they tend to be expensive, and many insurance providers may not offer coverage for their use in gender dysphoria. GnRH analogues are regarded as reversible. Should the patient desire to stop the medication, progression of their natal puberty would occur.

Limited outcome data exist regarding the use of puberty blockers. There are prospective studies that demonstrate a decrease in depressive symptoms and improvement in mental health outcomes. Many individuals who begin their journey with puberty blockers will continue with gender-affirming hormones later in life.

The GnRH analogues are not without side effects. Sex hormones play a vital role in bone mineral density deposition during the adolescent years. There is concern that prolonged use of puberty blockers may have a negative impact on bone development. Current evidence does not support a significant impact on bone development with short-term use, and bone accretion is observed with the initiation of gender-affirming hormones. Additionally, sex hormones may be important in neurocognitive function that develops during adolescence (Peper and Dahl 2013). Long-term studies on the use of GnRH analogues and their impact on bone mineral density, neurocognitive function, and mental health will be valuable in the years to come.

Starting Gender-Affirming Hormones

Gender-affirming hormones can promote both reversible and irreversible physiologic changes to the patient. Current criteria for gender-affirming hormones proposed by the WPATH Standards of Care (SOC v8) (2022) are (1) persistent, well-documented gender dysphoria; (2) capacity to make a fully informed decision and to give consent to treatment; (3) age of majority in their country; and (4) if significant medical or mental health concerns are present, they must be reasonably well controlled. Adolescent patients are not of the age of majority and always require consent from their parents or legal guardians unless emancipated. Due to the "semi-permanent" nature of gender-affirming hormones, the WPATH SOC v8 (2022) recommends a multidisciplinary approach to care that includes an evaluation by a skilled mental health provider. Such an evaluation can help affirm the diagnosis of gender dysphoria, identify goals of care, support that the patient can make an informed medical decision regarding their care, and verify there are no mental health issues that may cloud the individual's judgment regarding their care.

Transmasculine-Affirming Medications

Transmasculine individuals often desire the cessation of menses. For those who are not ready for testosterone therapy, therapeutic amenorrhea can be achieved by the use of combined hormone contraceptive pills. If there is strong opposition to estrogen-containing medications, then progesterone-only medications such as norethindrone or medroxyprogesterone can be very effective.

When testosterone is desired, attention must be taken to the patient's overall health and goals of care. Testosterone has the potential to cause birth defects, so testosterone is not appropriate for those who are pregnant or have the potential to become pregnant. In those who are engaging in receptive vaginal intercourse, the use of long-acting reversible hormonal contraceptives can be helpful to suppress menses and to prevent pregnancy in the setting of testosterone use. While testosterone is available in transdermal formulations, patients typically use injectable testosterone.

Testosterone can cause reversible and irreversible changes (Table 3.1). While many of these effects are desired masculine changes, some effects are not desired. It is important to discuss the potential of hair loss, acne, and weight gain with the patient and family. Further discussion regarding the uncertainty about fertility should also be discussed as fertility preservation may be desired (Fig. 3.1).

Testosterone should be used with caution in those with underlying liver disease, polycythemia, and coronary heart disease. The effects of testosterone on cardiovascular health are unknown in this population. Testosterone may promote poor cholesterol profiles, elevated blood pressure, or both. The Endocrine Society guidelines can assist with appropriate lab monitoring.

Table 3.1 Effects of testosterone regimen

Effect	Expected onset[a]	Expected maximum effect[a]
Skin oiliness/acne	1–6 months	1–2 years
Facial/body hair growth	3–6 months	3–5 years
Scalp hair loss	>12 months[b]	Variable
Increased muscle mass/strength	6–12 months	2–5 years[c]
Body fat redistribution	3–6 months	2–5 years
Cessation of menses	2–6 months	n/a
Clitoral enlargement	3–6 months	1–2 years
Vaginal atrophy	3–6 months	1–2 years
Deepened voice	3–12 months	1–2 years

Adapted with permission from Hembree et al. (2009). Copyright 2009, The Endocrine Society
Reprinted with permission from World Professional Association for Transgender Health (2022)
[a]Estimates represent published and unpublished clinical observations
[b]Highly dependent on age and inheritance; may be minimal
[c]Significantly dependent on the amount of exercise

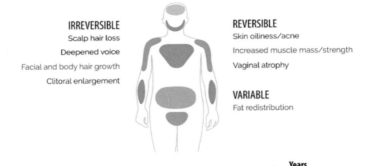

Fig. 3.1 Physical effects of masculinizing medications

Transfeminine-Affirming Medications

Transfeminine individuals have a variety of medical options available to promote feminization. The goal of medical interventions is twofold: (1) prevent undesired masculinization using an antiandrogen medication and (2) promote desired feminization by use of estradiol. It is important to discuss fertility preservation before starting feminizing medications.

There are a variety of antiandrogen options available to patients. Many individuals who were started on GnRH analogues as puberty blockers will often continue using these medications as an effective means to suppress androgen production. For those who may not have access to GnRH analogues, spironolactone, a potassium-sparing diuretic, has been used extensively in this population. Routine monitoring of electrolytes based on the Endocrine Society guidelines is appropriate with spironolactone use. The use of finasteride and progestins in this population is controversial and is not routinely recommended.

Estradiol is available in the form of an oral tablet, transdermal patch, and intramuscular injection. The feminizing effects of estradiol can be found in Table 3.2.

The risks of thrombosis with estradiol use have been described in detail for quite some time. It is important to perform a risk assessment on the patient, including asking about the personal history of smoking or blood clots and about the family history of blood clots and hormone-sensitive malignancies. The Endocrine Society provides detailed guidelines on laboratory monitoring of feminizing medications (Fig. 3.2).

Table 3.2 Effects of antiandrogen and estrogen regimen

Effect	Expected onset[a]	Expected maximum effect[a]
Body fat redistribution	3–6 months	2–5 years
Decreased muscle mass/strength	3–6 months	1–2 years[b]
Softening of skin/decreased oiliness	3–6 months	Unknown
Decreased libido	1–3 months	1–2 years
Decreased spontaneous erections	1–3 months	3–6 months
Male sexual dysfunction	Variable	Variable
Breast growth	3–6 months	2–3 years
Decreased testicular volume	3–6 months	2–3 years
Decreased sperm production	Variable	Variable
Thinning and slowed growth of body and facial hair	6–12 months	>3 years[c]
Male pattern baldness	No regrowth, loss stops 1–3 months	1–2 years

Adapted with permission from Hembree et al. (2009). Copyright 2009, The Endocrine Society
Reprinted with permission from World Professional Association for Transgender Health (2022)
[a]Estimates represent published and unpublished clinical observations
[b]Significantly dependent on amount of exercise
[c]Complete removal of male facial and body hair requires electrolysis, laser treatment, or both

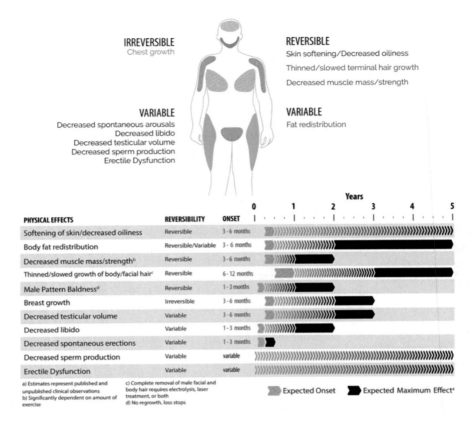

Fig. 3.2 Physical effects of feminizing medications

References

Delemarre-van de Waal HA, Cohen-Kettenis PT (2006) Clinical management of gender identity disorder in adolescents: a protocol on psychological and paediatric endocrinology aspects. Eur J Endocrinol 155(Suppl 1):131–137. https://doi.org/10.1530/eje.1.02231

Hembree WC, Cohen-Kettenis PT, Delemarre-van de Waal HA et al (2009) Endocrine treatment of transsexual persons: an endocrine society clinical practice guideline. J Clin Endocrinol Metab 94(9):3132–3154. https://doi.org/10.1210/jc.2009-0345

Hembree WC, Cohen-Kettenis PT, Gooren L et al (2017) Endocrine treatment of gender-dysphoric/gender-incongruent persons: an endocrine society clinical practice guideline. J Clin Endocrinol Metab 102(11):3869–3903. https://doi.org/10.1210/jc.2017-01658

Peper JS, Dahl RE (2013) Surging hormones: brain-behavior interactions during puberty. Curr Dir Psychol Sci 22(2):134–139. https://doi.org/10.1177/0963721412473755

World Professional Association for Transgender Health (WPATH) (2022) Standards of care for the health of transgender and gender diverse people, version 8. https://www.wpath.org/publications/soc

Chapter 4
Gender Affirmation: Surgical

Dana N. Johns, Emily M. Graham, and Cori A. Agarwal

Guidelines for Gender-Affirming Surgery

Although gender dysphoria in children does not commonly persist (Drummond et al. 2008; Wallien and Cohen-Kettenis 2008), adolescents with gender dysphoria often express pervasive feelings into adulthood (Steensma et al. 2013) (See Chap. 1 for definition of gender dysphoria). In fact, in a study by de Vries et al., 100% (70/70) of gender dysphoric adolescents given puberty-suppressing hormones went on to seek gender affirmation with hormone therapy, demonstrating the persistence of gender dysphoria with time (2011). Adolescents with gender dysphoria who receive early gender-affirming therapy also show improved psychological and functional outcomes when compared to baseline assessments (de Vries et al. 2014; The Lancet 2018). The treatment of gender dysphoric adolescents is complex and guided by recommendations from the World Professional Association for Transgender Health (WPATH) (2022). While the recommendations provided by WPATH are not strict requirements, they are followed by providers from various fields to provide the highest level of evidence-based care to gender dysphoric and gender-diverse individuals.

Treatment options for gender dysphoric adolescents fall under one of three treatment categories: fully reversible, partially reversible, and irreversible interventions. While the use of puberty blockers and hormone therapy are fully or partially reversible treatments, surgical interventions, including transmasculine and transfeminine

D. N. Johns (✉) · C. A. Agarwal
Division of Plastic Surgery, Department of Surgery, University of Utah, Salt Lake City, UT, USA
e-mail: dana.johns@hsc.utah.edu

E. M. Graham
Spencer Fox Eccles School of Medicine, University of Utah, Salt Lake City, UT, USA

top and bottom surgeries, are classified under irreversible interventions. While many of the WPATH guidelines for transgender adolescents are similar to those for adults, there are additional considerations for transgender adolescents including caregiver support and the capacity of the adolescent to provide informed consent. It is also important to note that not all adolescents with gender dysphoria will want to modify their bodies and that not all of those who choose to modify their bodies will want to modify their bodies to the same degree as another. Thus, decisions regarding treatment should always be patient-specific based on realistic goals of care with the support of a multidisciplinary healthcare team (Chen et al. 2016) with consideration of state laws for consent, which may vary by state.

Adolescent Transgender Surgical Overview

While multiple surgical procedures for gender affirmation are routinely performed on adult transgender individuals, the only gender-affirming surgery routinely performed on adolescents is masculinization of the chest (top surgery). This is partly because top surgeries are considered less ethically charged than bottom surgeries and because feminizing breast augmentations often require the use of feminization hormones to achieve positive cosmetic outcomes, whereas masculinizing chest creations can substitute hormone therapy with physical training to enhance the pectoralis and upper body musculature (Prior 2019; White Hughto and Reisner 2016). In addition to following WPATH guidelines, transgender adolescents seeking chest masculinization should obtain at least one referral letter from a mental health provider stating that the adolescent is mentally prepared and has the social support necessary to successfully receive gender-affirming surgery. Since many transgender adolescents seeking surgical treatment are already under the care of a skilled multidisciplinary team, obtaining a letter from a mental health provider trained to treat and refer an individual for surgery may not pose much difficulty. It is also recommended that the adolescent live in their identified gender for a minimum of 12 months. This will require the adolescent to come out to their family, friends, and those within their social network. This may present a challenge for those who do not live in affirming settings but will allow families and individuals the opportunity to experience daily life and family gatherings in the identified gender role.(Olson et. al. 2016) Once these suggested criteria are satisfied, obtaining a surgical consultation and plan of action is often straightforward. The following surgical overview in this section will focus on surgical considerations, technique and post-operative care, and complications for masculinizing top surgeries.

Preoperative Considerations

The initial consultation for gender-affirming masculinizing top surgery includes a complete history documenting the nature and extent of the gender dysphoria, a complete medical history, and a discussion about the goals and expectations of surgery.

Planning for postoperative social support is also an important part of the visit. Following the previously highlighted WPATH guidelines will facilitate this process.

As with any surgery, a healthy lifestyle reduces the risks of complications and optimizes results. Patients with obesity are encouraged to lose weight to lower their BMI to as close to 30 as possible; although a higher BMI does not preclude surgery, it may lead to poorer aesthetic results and potentially higher complications. Nicotine cessation is encouraged 4 weeks before and after surgery to improve wound healing and decrease infection complications. For patients on testosterone therapy, the aromatization of testosterone to estradiol theoretically increases the risk of perioperative venous thromboembolism (VTE). The extent of this risk is not well established, and the need to discontinue testosterone prior to chest surgery is controversial. Many surgeons do not require discontinuing testosterone but utilize sequential compression devices and early ambulation for VTE prophylaxis (Berry et al. 2012; Cregten-Escobar et al. 2012; Donato et al. 2017).

A thorough personal and family history of breast cancer is taken in all patients. Preoperative breast imaging is generally not obtained in adolescents unless family history or physical exam warrant it. For younger patients, the cost-benefit of sending the tissue to pathology is discussed, and a decision is made on a case-by-case basis. There are case reports of transgender men developing breast cancer after mastectomy (Burcombe et al. 2003; Nikolic et al. 2012; Vujovic et al. 2009), and it is important to discuss this with the patient before surgery and to council them that self-chest exams be continued throughout their life.

Selection of Surgical Technique

A variety of mastectomy techniques for transgender men have been described (Berry et al. 2012; Cregten-Escobar et al. 2012; Hage and Bloem 1995; Monstrey et al. 2008; Wolter et al. 2015). Choice of technique is based on multiple factors including breast size, degree of skin laxity, degree of ptosis, skin quality, and the size and position of the nipple-areolar complex (NAC). In selecting the technique, one must balance the desire to limit the extent of the scar with obtaining an optimal chest contour. The preferences of the patient regarding scars, willingness to undergo secondary and revision surgeries, and maintenance of NAC sensitivity are also factored into the technique selected.

Techniques can be broken down into three basic categories: the periareolar technique, a concentric circular technique with or without extended skin excision, and the "double incision" technique, usually with free nipple grafts. Adjunct procedures frequently performed include nipple reduction and liposuction.

While the periareolar mastectomy technique results in a small, well-hidden scar and typically maintains NAC sensation, its success relies on sufficiently small and non-ptotic breasts, small areolas, and good skin quality that will contract to the chest wall. Only a minority of patients, typically with small non-ptotic A cup breasts, are candidates for this technique (Fig. 4.1). In slightly larger breasts with a small amount of ptosis, additional skin excision patterns, most commonly a

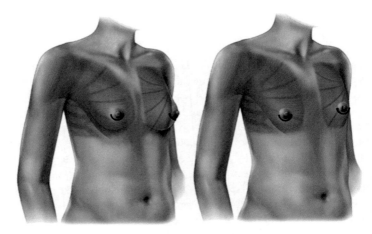

Fig. 4.1 Periareolar mastectomy technique. (Courtesy of Dana N. Johns, Cori A. Agarwal, and Emily M. Graham)

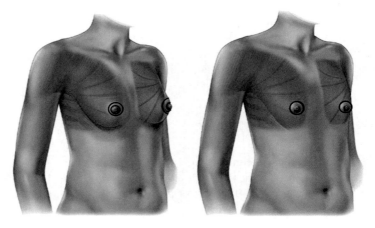

Fig. 4.2 Concentric circular mastectomy technique. (Courtesy of Dana N. Johns, Cori A. Agarwal, and Emily M. Graham)

concentric circular technique (Fig. 4.2), allow for excision of a small amount of skin and areolar reduction along with the mastectomy. NAC sensitivity is often maintained, but the revision rate is higher as flat contours are harder to ensure (Donato et al. 2017). For patients with larger breasts, moderate to severe ptosis, low positioned NACs, and poor skin quality, the best choice is the "double incision" mastectomy technique with free nipple grafting (Fig. 4.3). This technique creates reliable flap contours and optimal control over the size and position of the NAC on the chest wall. The primary disadvantage is the length of the scars and the loss of NAC sensation. All techniques require the placement of surgical drains and postoperative compression with a surgical vest.

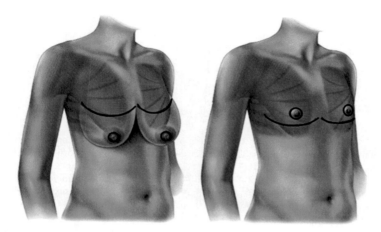

Fig. 4.3 Double incision mastectomy technique with free nipple grafting. (Courtesy of Dana N. Johns, Cori A. Agarwal, and Emily M. Graham)

Postoperative Care

A compression vest, drains, and, if applicable, the nipple graft pressure bolster are left in place for 1 week. At the first postoperative visit, the bolsters are removed and grafts and incisions inspected. Drains are removed once they are draining less than 30 milliliters (ml) per day, which is usually at the first visit. Patients will subsequently continue to wear their compression vest for a total of 4–6 weeks. During this time, patients have strict activity restrictions with minimal repetitive arm movements for 2–3 weeks and an additional 3 weeks of gradual increase in activity until they are released back to normal activity at 6 weeks from surgery.

Complications and Revisions

In the early postoperative period, hematoma is the most common complication, ranging from 5% to 15.4% (Berry et al. 2012; Cregten-Escobar et al. 2012; Donato et al. 2017; Kaariainen et al. 2017). The risk of hematoma formation is increased in patients undergoing periareolar techniques, likely due to the decreased visualization provided to the surgeon. Other acute complications include seroma formation and infection, which are usually able to be managed conservatively. Previous studies have shown NAC partial or complete loss as high as 2.3–17.9% (Bjerrome Ahlin et al. 2014; Colic and Colic 2000; Kaariainen et al. 2017).

The rate of revision surgery for chest reconstruction ranges considerably in the literature from 8% to 40% (Berry et al. 2012; Cregten-Escobar et al. 2012; Donato et al. 2017; Monstrey et al. 2008; Wolter et al. 2015). While some of these revisions may be planned, such as nipple or areolar reduction, other unplanned revisions include scar revisions, removal of residual excess skin, and dog ear excisions. Most revisions can be performed in the clinic under local anesthesia.

References

Berry MG, Curtis R, Davies D (2012) Female-to-male transgender chest reconstruction: a large consecutive, single-surgeon experience. J Plast Reconstr Aesthet Surg 65(6):711–719. https://doi.org/10.1016/j.bjps.2011.11.053

Bjerrome Ahlin H, Kolby L, Elander A et al (2014) Improved results after implementation of the Ghent algorithm for subcutaneous mastectomy in female-to-male transsexuals. J Plast Surg Hand Surg 48(6):362–367. https://doi.org/10.3109/2000656X.2014.893887

Burcombe RJ, Makris A, Pittam M et al (2003) Breast cancer after bilateral subcutaneous mastectomy in a female-to-male trans-sexual. Breast 12(4):290–293. https://doi.org/10.1016/s0960-9776(03)00033-x

Chen D, Hidalgo MA, Leibowitz S et al (2016) Multidisciplinary care for gender-diverse youth: a narrative review and unique model of gender-affirming care. Transgend Health 1(1):117–123. https://doi.org/10.1089/trgh.2016.0009

Colic MM, Colic MM (2000) Circumareolar mastectomy in female-to-male transsexuals and large gynecomastias: a personal approach. Aesthet Plast Surg 24(6):450–454. https://doi.org/10.1007/s002660010076

Cregten-Escobar P, Bouman MB, Buncamper ME et al (2012) Subcutaneous mastectomy in female-to-male transsexuals: a retrospective cohort-analysis of 202 patients. J Sex Med 9(12):3148–3153. https://doi.org/10.1111/j.1743-6109.2012.02939.x

de Vries AL, McGuire JK, Steensma TD et al (2014) Young adult psychological outcome after puberty suppression and gender reassignment. Pediatrics 134(4):696–704. https://doi.org/10.1542/peds.2013-2958

Donato DP, Walzer NK, Rivera A et al (2017) Female-to-male chest reconstruction: a review of technique and outcomes. Ann Plast Surg 79(3):259–263. https://doi.org/10.1097/SAP.0000000000001099

Drummond KD, Bradley SJ, Peterson-Badali M et al (2008) A follow-up study of girls with gender identity disorder. Dev Psychol 44(1):34–45. https://doi.org/10.1037/0012-1649.44.1.34

Hage JJ, Bloem JJ (1995) Chest wall contouring for female-to-male transsexuals: Amsterdam experience. Ann Plast Surg 34(1):59–66. https://doi.org/10.1097/00000637-199501000-00012

Kaariainen M, Salonen K, Helminen M et al (2017) Chest-wall contouring surgery in female-to-male transgender patients: a one-center retrospective analysis of applied surgical techniques and results. Scand J Surg 106(1):74–79. https://doi.org/10.1177/1457496916645964

Monstrey S, Selvaggi G, Ceulemans P et al (2008) Chest-wall contouring surgery in female-to-male transsexuals: a new algorithm. Plast Reconstr Surg 121(3):849–859. https://doi.org/10.1097/01.prs.0000299921.15447.b2

Murphy TF (2019) Adolescents and body modification for gender identity expression. Med Law Rev 27(4):623–639. https://doi.org/10.1093/medlaw/fwz006

Nikolic DV, Djordjevic ML, Granic M et al (2012) Importance of revealing a rare case of breast cancer in a female to male transsexual after bilateral mastectomy. World J Surg Oncol 10:280. https://doi.org/10.1186/1477-7819-10-280

Olson KR, Durwood L, DeMeules M et al (2016) Mental health of transgender children who are supported in their identities. Pediatrics 137(3):e20153223. https://doi.org/10.1542/peds.2015-3223

Prior JC (2019) Progesterone is important for transgender women's therapy-applying evidence for the benefits of progesterone in ciswomen. J Clin Endocr Metab 104(4):1181–1186. https://doi.org/10.1210/jc.2018-01777

Steensma TD, McGuire JK, Kreukels BP et al (2013) Factors associated with desistence and persistence of childhood gender dysphoria: a quantitative follow-up study. J Am Acad Child Adolesc Psychiatry 52(6):582–590. https://doi.org/10.1016/j.jaac.2013.03.016

The Lancet (2018) Gender-affirming care needed for transgender children. Lancet 391(10140):2576. https://doi.org/10.1016/S0140-6736(18)31429-6

Vujovic S, Popovic S, Sbutega-Milosevic G et al (2009) Transsexualism in Serbia: a twenty-year follow-up study. J Sex Med 6(4):1018–1023. https://doi.org/10.1111/j.1743-6109.2008.00799.x

Wallien MS, Cohen-Kettenis PT (2008) Psychosexual outcome of gender-dysphoric children. J Am Acad Child Adolesc Psychiatry 47(12):1413–1423. https://doi.org/10.1097/CHI.0b013e31818956b9

White Hughto JM, Reisner SL (2016) A systematic review of the effects of hormone therapy on psychological functioning and quality of life in transgender individuals. Transgend Health 1(1):21–31. https://doi.org/10.1089/trgh.2015.0008

Wolter A, Diedrichson J, Scholz T et al (2015) Sexual reassignment surgery in female-to-male transsexuals: an algorithm for subcutaneous mastectomy. J Plast Reconstr Aesthet Surg 68(2):184–191. https://doi.org/10.1016/j.bjps.2014.10.016

World Professional Association for Transgender Health (WPATH) (2022) Standards of Care for the Health of Transgender and Gender Diverse People, Version 8. https://www.wpath.org/publications/soc

Chapter 5
Related Clinical Issues

Lindsey Imber

Introduction

In addition to the gender-affirming medical and surgical issues discussed in previous chapters, two related areas that are important for transgender youth are gender-affirming voice therapy and nutritional care related to transgender medicine.

Gender-Affirming Voice Therapy

Brett Myers

Gender-affirming voice therapy is a service provided by a speech-language pathologist (SLP) who trains an individual to shape their voice and communication based on their personal goals. Therapy may address both verbal and nonverbal forms of communication. Verbal communication includes pitch, resonance, intonation, speech clarity, word choice, and other parameters. Nonverbal communication includes gesture, posture, facial expression, personal space, etc. All of these domains have the potential to convey gender, so the SLP will work with the individual to

Supplementary Information: The online version contains supplementary material available at https://doi.org/10.1007/978-3-031-18455-0_5.

L. Imber (✉)
Communication Sciences and Disorders, University of Utah, Salt Lake City, UT, USA

Nutrition Care Services, University of Utah, Salt Lake City, USA
e-mail: lindsey.imber@utah.edu

determine which items are important to address in therapy. Much like creating a homemade soup recipe, the individual has freedom to choose the ingredients that are likely to satisfy their goals. Adolescents may not be familiar with some of these concepts, so it is important for the SLP to teach the individual what each item means and how it can be linked to gender.

Because treatment is tailored to the individual, the duration of therapy is highly variable. It is often possible for some individuals to achieve their goals in several months of weekly visits, while others may need only a few weeks, and still others may need more time. The timeline of therapy is contingent upon the individual's familiarity with the concepts addressed, their pre-therapy abilities, and how frequently they are willing to practice and use their target voice outside of therapy. Anecdotally, adolescents seem to have more flexibility in their vocal expression than older adults, which assists them in adopting new vocal behaviors. When the individual feels confident and able to use their target voice in a variety of contexts-not only in the one-hour weekly therapy session-they tend to reach their goals more quickly.

Voice therapy can be beneficial for transfemales, transmales, and gender nonconforming individuals. Feminizing hormones have no effect on the voice, so voice therapy is traditionally a standard component of transfeminine care. Masculinizing hormones (specifically testosterone) typically deepen the pitch of the voice by adding mass to the vocal folds. Individuals who experience vocal changes from hormones can still benefit from behavioral voice therapy focused on other forms of communication outside of pitch.

If the voice does not match a person's gender identity, the individual may be subjected to misgendering by listeners and/or feelings of gender dysphoria (see Chap. 1 for definition of gender dysphoria). Therefore, the ultimate goal in voice therapy is to support the well-being and safety of the individual. To monitor progress toward an individual's goals, the SLP will periodically conduct acoustic and perceptual analyses, as well as assess client-reported outcomes via questionnaires. When both the client and clinician feel that all goals have been met, the individual will discontinue therapy and continue using the voice and communication techniques they developed independently. On occasion, individuals may return to the SLP for a follow-up visit to check maintenance of progress.

As examples of the changes resulting from voice therapy, Audio Files 1 and 2 were collected before and after a course of therapy for two patients: Jordan (18-year-old transgender male) and Alice (19-year-old transgender female).

Nutrition in Adolescent Transgender Medicine

Lindsey Imber

Guiding principles in nutrition assessment methods provide sex-based calculations and recommendations for calorie consumption and for macro- and micronutrient intake (U.S. Department of Health and Human Services 2020). Similarly, recommendations for body fat percentage, waist-hip ratio, and even Dietary Reference

Intakes (DRI) indicate distinctive values for males and females (National Academies of Sciences and Engineering n.d.). However, corresponding guidelines for transgender or gender non-conforming individuals do not exist. Sex-specific recommendations may not apply to gender non-conforming individuals. A notable gap in research limits knowledge of dietary intake needs and the validity and reliability of nutrition assessment methods and interventions for gender non-conforming individuals. Clinical judgment should guide nutrition recommendations based on gender identity. The discussion to follow reflects the clinical experience in the University of Utah Adolescent Medicine Clinic.

When considering nutrition for a transgender adolescent, it is important to remember that they are an adolescent first and foremost. Nutrition counseling for most adolescents begins with assessing current intake of key nutrients including protein, calcium, vitamin D, and hydration. Recommendations for transgender or gender non-conforming adolescents become more specific and individualized, based on the individual's gender journey. Treatment with puberty blockers (GnRH analogues), estrogen or testosterone, as well as surgery, will lead to specific recommendations.

When first meeting with an adolescent, it is best to start by building trust and rapport. This can be done by learning what the patient likes to do for fun, which may provide information about physical activity. Many adolescents do not participate in adequate physical activity, which may be exacerbated if they suffer from severe gender dysphoria and accompanying anxiety and depression (see Chap. 1 for definition of gender dysphoria). Moderate to vigorous physical activity becomes more challenging when an adolescent's body parts feel like they don't belong. Anxiety and depression can keep patients from being physically active because it can simply be overwhelming or they lose motivation. If this is the case, it is important to brainstorm activities that will provide movement but not exacerbate gender dysphoria or bring on symptoms of anxiety and to set goals that are manageable and can be completed even in the setting of depression. It is also important to note that transgender and gender non-conforming individuals are at an elevated risk for eating disorders and disordered eating patterns (Parker and Harriger 2020). Due to the strong influence mental health can have over one's relationship with food, it is crucial to also have a mental health provider as a part of the patient's care team.

Once the adolescent has become more comfortable sharing about themselves (which may not happen, presenting a bigger challenge) food can be discussed, beginning with a quick 24-hour recall. Adolescents may have difficulty describing what they eat, perhaps offering only that they eat certain meals. After reviewing the 24-hour recall, explore any food allergies/intolerances and foods that are disliked or avoided. This can provide insights into why certain foods do not appear in the recall and information on inadequate consumption of certain nutrients.

An in-depth discussion of each meal and snack should include generating ideas for tasty and healthy options. Many adolescents will report skipping breakfast due to time constraints. Brainstorming options for grab-and-go breakfasts that provide good, hearty nutrition can assist with goal setting. Sometimes adolescents will skip lunch as well because they don't like what's offered in the cafeteria or are uncomfortable eating at school. For those whose first "meal" of the day is an after-noon snack, emphasizing the importance of convenient healthy food (fruit in a bowl, veggie tray in the refrigerator, cheese sticks, etc.) rather than calorie dense "convenience foods" such as cookies, chips, and sugar-sweetened beverages is key.

Lunch discussion includes the options offered in the school cafeteria for those who purchase/receive school lunch. Brainstorming options and combinations can be essential to the adolescent getting a nutritious lunch at school. If they pack their lunch, it is important to come up with ideas for healthy lunches that taste good and don't take too much time to prepare. For most adolescents, taste trumps nutrients, so it is crucial to find healthy foods and preparation methods that appeal to the youth's taste buds.

After lunch, dinner is discussed. It is important to ask if family dinner is something that happens in their household, if the adolescent assists in preparing dinner, and if they enjoy cooking. Dinner seems to be the easiest meal to manipulate because usually it is the meal in which the parents are the most involved.

Next, it is time to discuss snacks and beverages. Encourage snacks that combine protein and fruits or vegetables, such as peanut butter and an apple or celery. Beverages are discussed with a focus on the challenge of excess consumption of sugar-sweetened beverages. Suggesting flavored sparkling water and other beverages that are not sweetened with sugar and still appeal to adolescent can be helpful.

After diet and exercise are discussed, education needs are evaluated. Education for most adolescents is general and begins with the healthy plate. Most adolescents have already seen examples of the healthy plate, also known as MyPlate (U.S. Department of Agriculture n.d.), so a good starting place is asking them what they know about it. Then discuss each category individually, reviewing foods in that category and their importance to body functions and health. Start with the fruit and vegetable portion, which takes up 50% of the plate. Most adolescents know what fruits and vegetables are, so this discussion is brief. It is important to note that fruits and vegetables hold nutrients that are essential to body function. Without these nutrients, body function can decline over time, but isn't noticed right away. This is why it is important to make sure fruits and vegetables are eaten on a regular basis; they provide long-term nutrition. Then follow with protein, including plant-based options. Finally, discuss carbohydrates and the difference between simple and complex carbohydrates. Emphasizing the balance of the three categories can be easier than having youth focus on the foods they "need to eat" or "need to avoid."

The first, and often biggest, challenge for most adolescents is adequate consumption of fruits and vegetables, which is particularly hard at breakfast. Protein intake is second, usually lacking at breakfast and throughout the day. Consuming simple carbohydrates is more convenient and often the chosen option. Suggesting combining a protein food and a fiber food (whole grain/fruit/vegetable) at all meals and snacks may be useful. Bring attention to creating a balanced diet with the "healthy plate" recommended portion sizes, variety, and key nutrients.

Past this point, education becomes more individualized; including an understanding of metabolism and how hormones affect it can be helpful. Although research is limited on gender identity-specific nutrition, hormone therapy can change metabolic needs. Masculinizing or feminizing hormone therapy may cause altered blood pressure, changes in lipid and glucose levels, weight gain, and changes in appetite, body, and bone composition (Seal 2016). When a patient first starts their gender journey, they may take hormone (or puberty) blockers. The dietitian's job is to discuss how those may affect health and teach how this can be mitigated with diet. When a patient starts medications that block reproductive hormones (puberty blockers or anti-androgens), it is important to focus on bone health, including discussion of calcium, vitamin D, and weight-bearing physical activity. Emphasize that appropriate consumption of these nutrients, along with being physically active, will help to ensure they achieve optimal physical health.

For transfemales taking estrogen, nutrition education is focused on bone health and on how healthy eating and exercise can have a positive effect on bones. For transmales taking testosterone, education on the role of protein and exercise (strength training exercises in particular) in muscle building and lipid profiles is provided. For these patients, creating a balanced diet is important as well. Testosterone can affect appetite and increase cravings, so discussing healthy snack options that have a protein and fiber pairing as well as encouraging regular exercise is vital.

When a patient is considering surgery, pre- and postsurgery nutrition is discussed. This is the same for any patient regardless of gender or sex. A standard increase in typical calorie and protein consumption is recommended for wound healing. It is important to consume the proper amount of calories and protein as well as a good variety of foods to provide key nutrients both before and after surgery to decrease recovery time and improve outcomes (Arnold and Barbul 2006).

Overall, education and goal setting are the most important components of nutrition counseling for transgender adolescents. It is imperative to have the adolescent involved in setting goals; understanding motivation for change will assist in goal setting and guide recommendations. Education should be individualized, based on the adolescent's background and their gender journey goals. Let the adolescent guide what is important and manageable for them. Creating a healthy, well-balanced plate and maintaining appropriate activity levels should always be a focus.

Acknowledgments The author thanks Brett Myers, PhD, CCC-SLP, for the contribution to Chap. 5.

References

Arnold M, Barbul A (2006) Nutrition and wound healing. Plast Reconstr Surg 117 (7 Suppl):42S–58S. https://doi.org/10.1097/01.prs.0000225432.17501.6c. PMID: 16799374.
National Academies of Sciences and Engineering (n.d.) Food and Nutrition Board Publications. https://www.nationalacademies.org/fnb/food-and-nutrition-board
Parker LL, Harriger JA (2020) Eating disorders and disordered eating behaviors in the LGBT population: a review of the literature. J Eat Disord 8, 51. https://doi.org/10.1186/s40337-020-00327-y

Chapter 6
Equity and Inclusivity

Nicole L. Mihalopoulos

Creating a Safe and Inclusive Environment for Transgender and Gender-Diverse Individuals

Historically, institutions have not been affirming to transgender and gender-diverse individuals. This is problematic as years of oppression and failure of these institutions to promote inclusion and equity have fostered distrust in transgender/gender-diverse individuals of academic institutions and medical systems. For example, a transgender man may avoid seeking care for acute abdominal pain due to past negative experiences at an emergency room, starting with the registration staff and forms he had to complete to the language used (not asking preferred name and pronouns) and the physical examination by the physician. Clinical research historically fails to include transgender/gender-diverse individuals, not until 2015 did the National Institutes of Health (NIH) establish the Sexual and Gender Minority Research Office (NIH 2022). It is up to everyone, from frontline staff to researchers to executive leadership, to identify these inequities and promote a safe, affirming, and inclusive environment.

N. L. Mihalopoulos (✉)
Division of Adolescent Medicine, Department of Pediatrics, University of Utah,
Salt Lake City, UT, USA
e-mail: nicole.mihalopoulos@hsc.utah.edu

© The Author(s), under exclusive license to Springer Nature Switzerland AG 2022   37
A. W. Dell et al., *Providing Affirming Care to Transgender and Gender-Diverse Youth*, SpringerBriefs in Public Health, https://doi.org/10.1007/978-3-031-18455-0_6

Staff Education

Support staff are typically the first people encountered at a healthcare visit. The initial impression they provide will often set the tone for the rest of the visit. A variety of tool kits are available to help with staff training to promote a safe and affirming environment (Advocates for Youth 2020; GLSEN 2019).

Signage

Consider adding signs around the facility that demonstrate support for transgender and gender-diverse youth. Seeing the blue/pink/white colors (Fig. 6.1) on a sign or a lapel pin can help individuals recognize that they are in a safe environment.

Language

Using inclusive language is essential. Do not assume that individuals are male or female based on appearance. Do not assume that individuals are in a relationship with an opposite-sex partner. Starting conversations with "How would you like to be called?" and "What are your pronouns?" are great ways to set the tone for encounters. Using terms like "Tell me about your partner" instead of "Do you have a girlfriend?" can minimize risk of making either party uncomfortable.

Forms/Electronic Medical Record

Some healthcare systems and electronic medical records (EMRs) integrate an individual's desired name or pronouns. Providers can advocate to expand EMRs to include preferred gender, legal gender, sex assigned at birth, and sexual identity. For

Fig. 6.1 Transgender sign

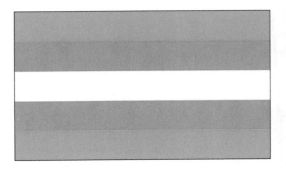

transgender and gender-diverse individuals, updating the patient's organ inventory (e.g., uterus, ovaries, prostate, testicles) as part of the preventive health measure checklist can often be helpful to ensure healthcare maintenance is being properly addressed (e.g., transmasculine individuals may need cervical cancer screening or breast cancer screening). However, asking, "What parts do you have?" is inappropriate at a visit for such things as an ear infection or ingrown toenail. Using a gender identity two-step approach on intake forms can be affirming to patients and can promote an inclusive environment:

Gender Identity (Two-Step)
1. What is your gender identity?
   - ☐ Male
   - ☐ Female
   - ☐ Transgender man / transman
   - ☐ Transgender woman / transwoman
   - ☐ Genderqueer / gender non-conforming
   - ☐ Additional identity (fill in) _____
   - ☐ Decline to state
2. What sex were you assigned at birth?
   - ☐ Male
   - ☐ Female
   - ☐ Decline to state

Advertising/Marketing

It is important for businesses and medical establishments with initiatives that promote inclusion to market themselves to the target population. Transgender and gender-diverse youth seek settings in which they will feel safe. In addition to welcoming signage and communications training for frontline staff, businesses and medical establishments can add "LGBTQ-friendly" or "Transgender Safe Space" attributes on their Google business web page. Larger institutions should consider adopting policies, practices, and benefits to achieve the Corporate Equality Index (Human Rights Campaign 2021) or Healthcare Equality Index (Human Rights Campaign 2020) as designated by the Human Rights Campaign.

Advocacy and Policies

Support from Family and Healthcare Providers

The Endocrine Society (Hembree et al. 2017) and the World Professional Association for Transgender Health (2022) provide guidelines for the provision of medical and surgical gender-affirming care for transgender children, adolescents, and adults.

Both organizations recommend that parents/guardians/families support children and adolescents in social gender role transition. In the case that a family does not allow a child to make a gender-role transition, healthcare providers should counsel families to support their child in a nurturing way that allows the child to explore gender feelings and behavior in a safe environment. An example of supporting children in the home is to use the name and pronouns preferred by the child.

Providers may find additional information in the position statement from three professional organizations with members that provide care to children and adolescents. The Human Rights Campaign Foundation along with the American Academy of Pediatrics and the American College of Osteopathic Pediatricians published "Supporting and Caring for Transgender Children" (Human Rights Campaign 2016). This document emphasizes the importance of initiating gender-affirming care during childhood when appropriate, rather than "watchful waiting" until a child is 18 years of age (and able to provide consent without parents). The Association of American Family Physicians recommends that "adolescents experiencing puberty should be evaluated for reversible puberty suppression, which may make future affirmation easier and safer. Aspects of affirming care should not be delayed until gender stability is ensured. Multidisciplinary care may be optimal but is not universally available" (Klein et al. 2018, pp. 645). It is also recommended that clinicians read the *Code of Medical Ethics* published by the American Medical Association (2021) and review relevant recommendations regarding population care.

Pediatric healthcare providers have a greater responsibility to advocate on behalf of their patients because children cannot vote and need a voice to protect their access to health care. Additionally, pediatricians can write letters to support changes in legal documents that are congruent with an individual's lived gender, to improve insurance coverage of transgender health care (especially for puberty blockers and surgery) and access to gender-affirming restrooms and locker rooms in schools.

State/National Advocacy

Healthcare providers can advocate for their patients locally and nationally by working with policymakers to create laws that provide for equality in healthcare access. Equality includes health insurance benefits that pay for services related to medical and surgical gender-affirming care and mental health services. Further advocacy may include housing, employment, and anti-discrimination laws. Table 6.1 describes several national advocacy organizations that seek to create equality for sexual and gender minorities. Additionally, each state has an equality organization that advocates for the equal rights of its citizens. Here are a few of them:

- Arizona—Equality Arizona (equalityarizona.org)
- New Hampshire—Freedom New Hampshire (freedomnewhampshire.org)
- Missouri—PROMO (promoonline.org)
- South Dakota—Equality South Dakota (www.eqsd.org)
- Utah—Equality Utah (www.equalityutah.org)

Table 6.1 National organizations that advocate for transgender equality

Organization	Description
GLAAD (glaad.org)	Works through entertainment, news, and digital media to share stories from the LGBTQ+ community that accelerate acceptance. Originally title "Gay and Lesbian Alliance Against Defamation," the organization changed its name to GLAAD in 2013 in order to incorporate bisexual and transexual individuals as well as allies from diverse backgrounds
Human Rights Campaign (www.hrc.org)	Supports political campaigns, individuals, and institutions via a set of comprehensive programs focused on mobilizing those who advocate for LGBTQ+ equality. Resources specific to youth include: Supporting & Caring for Transgender Children (www.hrc.org/resources/supporting-caring-for-transgender-children) Welcoming Schools (welcomingschools.org) Project THRIVE: A National Campaign to Support LGBTQ Youth (www.thehrcfoundation.org/professional-resources/project-thrive) Time to Thrive annual national conference (timetothrive.org)
National Center for Transgender Equality (transequality.org)	Advocates to change policies and society to increase understanding and acceptance of transgender people
PFLAG (pflag.org)	The first and largest organization for lesbian, gay, bisexual, transgender, and queer (LGBTQ+) people, their parents and families, and allies. Chapters across the U.S. further the mission of equality through online learning programs, advocacy support, media training, and community service projects to name a few. Originally known as "Parents, Families, and Friends of Lesbians and Gays," the organization changed its name to simply PFLAG in 2014 to include all individuals on the broader spectrum of sexuality and gender diversity
Transgender Law Center (transgenderlawcenter.org)	Advocates for policy research and development and assists with litigation in areas such as employment, education, housing, immigration, and health care, challenging the legal system to respect the dignity and humanity of transgender and gender nonconforming individuals

References

Advocates for Youth (2020) Creating safer spaces for LGBTQ youth: A toolkit for education, healthcare, and community-based organizations. https://www.advocatesforyouth.org/resources/curricula-education/creating-safer-spaces-for-lgbtq-youth

American Medical Association (2021) Code of medical ethics overview. https://www.ama-assn.org/delivering-care/ethics/code-medical-ethics-overview

GLSEN (2019) The safe space kit: A guide to supporting lesbian, gay, bisexual, transgender, and queer students in your school. https://www.glsen.org/activity/glsen-safe-space-kit-solidarity-lgbtq-youth

Hembree WC, Cohen-Kettenis PT, Gooren L et al (2017) Endocrine treatment of gender-dysphoric/gender-incongruent persons: an endocrine society clinical practice guideline. J Clin Endocrinol Metab 102(11):3869–3903. https://doi.org/10.1210/jc.2017-01658

Human Rights Campaign (2016) Supporting & caring for transgender children. Human Rights Campaign, Washington, D.C.

Human Rights Campaign (2020) Healthcare Equality Index 2020. https://www.hrc.org/resources/
 healthcare-equality-index
Human Rights Campaign (2021) Corporate Equality Index 2021. https://www.hrc.org/resources/
 corporate-equality-index
Klein DA, Paradise SL, Goodwin ET (2018) Caring for transgender and gender-diverse persons:
 what clinicians should know. Am Fam Physician 98(11):645–653
National Institutes of Health (NIH) (2022) Sexual & Gender Minority Research Office. https://
 dpcpsi.nih.gov/sgmro
World Professional Association for Transgender Health (WPATH) (2022) Standards of care
 for the health of transgender and gender-diverse people, version 8. https://www.wpath.org/
 publications/soc

Index

Printed in the United States
by Baker & Taylor Publisher Services